PRAISE FOR HARRIET CABELLY

"No life is exempt from suffering, and therefore each and every one of us could benefit greatly from learning to turn pain into purpose. Harriet Cabelly's journey provides inspiration, encouragement, and a compass that can guide us towards the light and help us grow through hardship."

Tal Ben-Shahar, Founder Happiness Studies Academy

"When we enter new and challenging territory, a guide who knows it well is what we need most. Harriet is a wonderful guide for any of us facing cancer and all that it brings."

Rabbi Steve Leder, NY Times Bestselling Author

"To find the miracle in the day, we must first be present to the possibility of doing so. Through clear, honest, warm and engaging moments, Harriet Cabelly models for us the potency of remaining awake to the good that may occur, even in the presence of illness,

even when life is on the line. Moreover, we are gifted, through her mindful experience, practices and perspectives that may ground any one of us in what we can control when darkness rises. Her tale is a tale of resilience in action, of a robust spirit and generous heart, unafraid to both face death and embrace life."

Maria Sirois, author of *A Short Course in Happiness After Loss (and Other Dark, Difficult Times)*

"A personal journey through a cancer diagnosis, celebrating moments of joy and highlighting ways to cope."

Delia Ephron, author of *Left on Tenth: A Second Chance at Life*

LIGHT THROUGH

Darkness

Miracles along
my Cancer Journey

HARRIET CABELLY

Red Penguin
BOOKS

Light Through Darkness

Copyright © 2024 by Harriet Cabelly

All rights reserved.

Published by Red Penguin Books

Bellerose Village, NY

Library of Congress Control Number: 2024927024

ISBN

Digital 978-1-63777-677-3

Print 978-1-63777-678-0 | 978-1-63777-679-7

To my most dedicated, committed, steadfast,

fun-loving and silly hubby

who travelled this journey with me 24/7.

CONTENTS

"There are only two ways to live your life. One is as though nothing is a miracle. The other is as though everything is a miracle."

ALBERT EINSTEIN

MY STORY

I was taken up to my room alone after hearing the words, "large mass sitting on three major organs." Hubby was not allowed to come up with me at 11 PM post covid. Tears flowing uncontrollably, he was told to go home and come back the next morning. How he managed to safely drive home to Long Island from Lenox Hill Hospital in the city is a miracle. Tears like that are vision blockers; and mini eye-glass windshield wipers that as kids we all said we'd invent, wouldn't have done it anyways. These tears were coming from deep within the heart of the body.

Into a dark room that certainly matched my astonishingly horrific news, the waiting nurse greeted me by asking if there was anything more I needed besides the turned down blanket, propped up pillows and directions to the remote on the bed. "Yes," I wanted to scream, "I want to go home. I only came in for fluids for dehydration."

That Sunday morning, March of 2022, I went to the boardwalk at Long Beach to see if my nourishing and favorite place by the ocean waves would help me feel better. Little did I know that hours later the waves of my life would come crashing down. But after a couple of minutes, my legs wouldn't carry me as they always did through the 4.2 miles of roundtrip boardwalk. I had to sit down on the bench. Not so terrible as it faced the water to one of my favorite sounds of waves. But yes, it was terrible as something was very wrong with this avid walker.

I must be dehydrated was all hubby Alan and I could figure. I really didn't want to go to the emergency room but a call with my trainer friend, Mitch, echoed the need to just go and get some fluids.

After speaking with my son-in-law's uncle who had been the head of gastroenterology at Lenox Hill Hospital, we drove to their ER. On some level, I sensed if the need arose and I had to be admitted, he'd connect me with a good doctor.

"What are you here for" the triage nurse asked. "I'm probably dehydrated since I feel very weak, so I came for fluids." Quiet and empty on this Sunday afternoon, I was taken in quickly. After telling the ER doctor my stomach issues of the past few months, she suggested I have a CT scan. "But I had one pretty recently, a little over a year ago and it was fine; and I just had an endoscopy a few months ago and that was basically fine short of some gastritis and h-pylori which was taken care of." I eventually yielded to her lovely manner and instruction that I need not finish the whole bottle of the pre-CT scan light-up drink.

After being told the scan results would take about an hour, I relaxed back on the bed up against the wall in my tiny curtained-off area. Hubby and I joked and laughed as I flashed my exposed tushy walking to the bathroom wearing that silly back-side open hospital gown.

The no-news is good news line doesn't always hold up. This evening, the no-news after an hour meant more bathroom trips out of sheer worry and not knowing what to do with myself, more questions to the nursing station of "did they forget about me," and eventually after almost three hours, the appearance of an unknown woman to my makeshift room.

I already didn't like what I saw: a new person coming my way. Where was my ER doctor? Then again, where had she been the whole time I was waiting, never coming by to say anything during the anxiety-provoking wait. A changing of the guard, as I was told. The ER staff shift had changed and now I was being addressed by a new young doctor who quickly explained how bad she felt not knowing me at all and having to tell me these results. Uh oh, heart beating as fast as possible without popping out of my chest. "The results of the scan show a large mass sitting on three main organs. More testing must be done." I felt myself harden against the wall, stone-like in stature, numb in feeling and body and heart completely disconnected. "How were they talking about me. I just had a great tango lesson three days earlier, on Thursday, and I have a video to show for it," I thought. For hubby, who was standing near me, no amount of tears could put out this fire. For me, not one salty reminder of the earlier waves fell. All I heard was the prediction of death – an end to my 67-year-old love of life. Clearly there wasn't much more to clarify from this doctor. "You will be admitted and taken up to a room for more testing in the next few days, but being it's past visiting hours, he can't go upstairs with you; he can come back tomorrow. I'm very sorry."

She left and I turned to Alan and what came out of my mouth was, "if this is really the case and I'm dying, I want to go into hospice. No treatment!." In his calm way, he said, "let's not talk about this now; we don't know anything for sure yet." But I needed him to know my wishes and I felt very clear in them. I did not want to go through awful sickness from the treatment if I had only a short time left.

Drop a possible death sentence and within minutes we each go our separate ways. Somewhere along the way to my room, my heart fell off that gurney and I felt myself being wheeled into oblivion.

I had never been hospitalized except for the times I gave birth to each of my three daughters. The good reason for being in a hospital, the healthy reason. And now in the seconds of being told bad news, I became a sick patient. Propped up in bed I started thinking, "How is this even possible? I exercise every day, meditate a few times a week, gave up junk and processed food and most refined sugars years ago, live with purpose and enthusiasm, have good friends and have strong faith. These are actually most of the ingredients of the Blue Zones, the places in the world where people live the healthiest and longest. Oh, and no small fact of important genetics here: my parents lived into their upper 90s, never having had cancer."

"How is this happening to me?!!!!!!" The bitter salt started coming down with a vengeance.

The 'why me' began to knock softly.

I had worked on this 'why me' many years ago when my middle daughter, Nava, was diagnosed with agenesis of the corpus collosum at ten months old, a neurological problem where the mid-section of the brain that divides the right and left hemispheres does not fully develop in the first trimester. She would have lifelong disabilities, the extent of which was not known at that point. I went into a tailspin of intense negative feelings. My bitterness and anger sent me to a therapist's office where I vented with rage and grief wanting to comprehend how such an unexpected tragedy could happen. Was this a punishment? Had I done something so bad to warrant such pain with what would be forever: raising a child with disabilities? As Ken, my wonderful therapist explained to me, "you are grieving the loss of the perfect child; the loss of a shattered dream." And all I could focus on was why this happened to my child, to me.

With all my searching in books, both Jewish and secular, and in therapy, there were no 'real' answers to the 'why me' question. It was a futile exercise in existential philosophy that could be debated forever, as to 'why bad things happen to good people.'

My work was giving up the struggle of trying to make sense of this awfulness, and moving in the direction of beginning to act upon my new reality. He was guiding me towards the 'how' and 'what' concepts. 'Why' would just keep me in a dark hole at the bottom of a deep cave, flailing my arms screaming 'help, I don't understand why I'm down here.' It wouldn't do anything to help me start my climb back up and out into the light. 'What' and 'how' would help me begin to figure out how to handle the situation I was now in and what I needed to do to climb up and not remain stuck in the bottom of the muck of angst and resentment.

My year in therapy set me on a better course. The intense feelings of grief loosened their grip around my neck so I could breathe a little easier and feel a bit lighter. I could now go to the playground with other babies and toddlers running all over without feeling such jealousy and bitterness, while my little Nava sat smiling placidly in her stroller.

My then-husband and I came to our parenting mission for Nava: we would parent her towards independence. This became our guiding light, our compass directing us towards helping her develop a strong sense of self - confidence and self-pride - in her progress and developing abilities. When Nava was finally starting to walk at age three, and did the typical fall downs, I stopped myself from running over to pick her up and watched her struggle to get back up on her own. And each time she did it, we applauded and said "yay, you did it" and she beamed that big Navi smile. That carried into much of her learning. So much so that today, at age 42, if I want to do banking for her, she says, "no, I can go myself and the teller will help me figure out how to put my new card in to withdraw my money." And pride swells my heart and wetness fills my eyes.

Back in my dark hospital room, my roommate snoring away, the stop sign of 'why me' goes up in my mind so as to prevent those poisonous words from entering my bloodstream. I did not want it sucking the life out of me, whatever life I had left. I did not want to go into that dark cave again flailing to get out. Bitterness was not to be my pill of choice.

As exhaustion set in, my kids, all adults now, came to mind. They are all on their own, high functioning in their own lives – a most rewarding legacy. And my own life, rich and gratifying,

staying closely engaged in all that is meaningful and important to me, pursuing new experiences, taking on new goals and
interests, a curious lover of learning and living life in awe of all
its beauty and wonderment; and yes, dealing and growing
through painful difficulties. And always a bit melancholy as
the bright light of day starts to fade, another day never to be
had again; and always happy when I wake up and go to my
window to see the sky start to streak with soft colors
announcing itself, "I'm here again, and you're here with me."

I realized I wasn't scared of dying; I just wanted more life,
more living time. I did not want my time to be up yet. Like a
rose's petals dropping, my tears began to fall softly and gently,
as I finally drifted off to sleep.

PART ONE

THE TEN MIRACLES

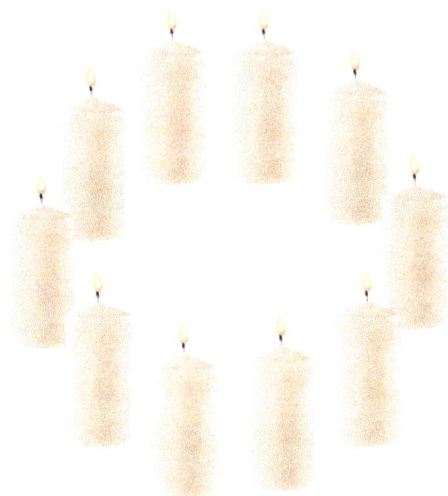

THE MIRACLE OF LIFE RENEWED
THE FIRST MIRACLE

That first week went by with tests, biopsies and stents put in to open up my bile ducts as they were being blocked. "Didn't you see your eyes were yellow," the ER nurse asked. "No!" I didn't see yellow in my eyes or that sickly color anywhere on my skin. My bilirubin numbers had quickly gone sky-high from two weeks earlier when I had blood work done and they were normal. To prevent my liver from shutting down, two stents were inserted through an advanced type of endoscopy.

A social worker was sent to my room, who I found out was from palliative care. I immediately made known to her my wishes of wanting to go into hospice. "If my diagnosis ends up being what they thought in the ER on Sunday night, I don't want treatment." There, now I had said it out loud to two people. It was becoming more real.

I don't know how I dealt my way through until Saturday, six days later from that life-altering ER declaration and 4-day hospital stay, thinking my end was in sight. Saturday was the day I got my official diagnosis. But I didn't know that when I lit my Sabbath candles on Friday evening at sundown. I said the blessings over the candles praying for the best possible outcome and the strength to deal with it, knowing the call was pending anytime with the results of the biopsies.

Saturday is the Jewish Sabbath and I observe it. It has always brought me great comfort to welcome it in at the end of a hectic week. I light my Sabbath candles and plop down on the couch with a great sigh of relief, feeling the lightness of the next 24-hour day settle into my bones; a day off from busyness. The Sabbath cuts a clear demarcation line between the five weekdays and this day of rest and relaxation. It lights the way towards a complete difference in the space of time and energy. Time takes on a different essence. It's more of being, less of doing. I pile my books and other reading material on my coffee table, looking forward to slowly turning the pages without a time limit or guilt feeling of what 'needs' to be done. The list of things to do gets put off until after sundown on Saturday night.

This Sabbath I obviously felt anything but relief. Normally I don't answer the phone as Saturday is unplug-from-all day. But I knew I would be answering this one.

At our Sabbath lunch, after morning prayers usually at synagogue but that morning at home, our good friends, Susan and Richie stopped by. I don't know how I choked down any food in that waiting space of terror. The phone finally rang. It was Dr. Benais, the interventionist gastro doctor who had placed my two stents, with the news that the biopsies showed it was lymphoma. I quickly gave the phone to Richie who's a podiatrist and therefore understands the medical jargon and had him further talk to the doctor. I could not focus and take it all in, nor could hubby.

Within minutes after that call came the one that put me on a better course. Myron, the family gastro doctor who had referred me to Lenox Hill Hospital and gotten this great doctor, called and said, "I have good news; if you have to have cancer, this is one of the better ones to have – non-Hodgkin's lymphoma – known to have a very good prognosis." There I had it, my official diagnosis. A far cry from the initial preliminary one.

Death sentence averted!

This was certainly not the life-sentence cancer that had revealed itself in the ER when I was told a very large mass was sitting on three major organs. I took it as if that's the case, I didn't want to be sick from treatment in the short time I had left.

There is a period between the Jewish holidays of Rosh Hashanah and Yom Kippur known as the Ten Days of Repentance or the Days of Awe (Yamim Nora'im), a time of inner reflection and repentance. We ask for forgiveness and look inward to our thoughts, feelings and behaviors. We hope and pray for renewal and a good outcome to our asking. On Rosh Hashanah our fate is written down for the coming year; on Yom Kippur it is sealed. In between, those 10 days, is a serious time of decision-making by G-d.

My verdict was changed that week. Although it was not this holiday season, I feel that my week was book-ended between these two holy and important days. And that G-d changed His mind from an awful decree to a better one and decided to save my life.

THE MIRACLE OF SANCTUARY
THE SECOND MIRACLE

My oncologist who came highly recommended as someone on the cutting edge of research in lymphoma was at Columbia Presbyterian hospital. I questioned the idea of not going to Memorial Sloan Kettering hospital as that is known as one of the best cancer hospitals, but I was told, "you go where the best doctor for your particular cancer is." And so Columbia was to be my hospital of treatment and care.

My referring doctor, Myron, strongly advised me to go through their emergency room to be admitted instead of waiting a couple of weeks to have my first appointment with the oncologist. He was clearly very concerned. On the following Sunday night, a week later from my life-changing ER experience, I had another awful time in Columbia's ER. Not the kind where you sit for hours on end waiting to be seen. Rather where you lay in-waiting in an area with no curtain of separation from your partner patient, especially in the close aftermath of Covid. I was grateful my partner was not retching or throwing up as

I've had an aversion and fear of vomiting for as long as I can remember. Nobody came in to check on me, or offer drink or food, nothing. The only thing I got was a rough high-up swab in the nose for Covid soon after I got into my bed.

Once you know things are running amuck in your body, you want to get going on treating those rascals. And so ruminating and watching the large clock's hands move throughout the wee hours of the night were my all-nighter activities. Sleep had barely visited my body and mind. When morning finally came, I figured maybe the changing of the shift would create some attention and movement. The entire time hubby had been out there 'almost' yelling (as screaming is not his nature), he was told there's not enough staff and they knew in advance I was not a critical case right now.

Finally someone came in to wheel me out. I thought I was being taken to my room but no, I was wheeled to another area-in-waiting. This time though it was a private tiny walled in space with a bathroom right near. Step one – yay, we were getting closer!

And now to the best part where I was finally taken up to my room. I was wheeled into a ...... drumroll here.... a private room with one deep purple wall and a water view! What a surprising reward after my nightmarish experience in the ER. It was as if this room had my name on it. I could actually say I was so excited when I came through the door. My visual senses came alive as I felt embraced by beauty that felt personal to me, as if to beckon me in with, "now here's your purple and here's your view."

Now you need to know something here so as to appreciate this sight for very sore and sleepy eyes: purple is and has been my favorite color since I was sixteen. When I finally got my own room back then, my mom and I picked out a deeply rich shade of purple plush shag carpet and velvet bed cover. I recall that as being the start of my great purple appeal. And my love for it has grown along with me. I am known as the purple person and am therefore a very easy person to buy a gift for; along with my being a giraffe lover. I used to dream about opening a café or bookstore called the Purple Giraffe.

I am also a nature lover. Water has always been a soothing balm for me. It's expansive, reflective of light in its various forms, deep and has lots of movement. It draws you in, if not physically, then mentally and emotionally. It takes me to a place of calm. To have a view of the Hudson River (on the west side of Manhattan) was a piece of tranquility as I would breathe in moments of ease. The nurses were so attentive and accommodating that they helped me rearrange the furniture with my bed practically lying up against the window so that my eyes and mind's focus was on the water more than on the hospital room. And the piece de resistance was that I could ooh and ahh over the painted canvas each night of oranges, pinks and lavenders that ended the day in all its beauty. What an uplift to the pallor of sickness.

I soon learned that this very private area that was kept locked, was a newly designed unit aimed at healing and tranquility, and was reserved for patients receiving stem cell transplants. I was put here because their regular cancer floor unit was full.

A miracle of a room!

And this was where I first met my oncologist – another oasis within difficulties. As I came out of my bathroom I was greeted by a young woman with long dark straight hair, a beautiful summery dress and heels. Who was this person who matched this beautiful room, who looked like she stepped out of Vogue magazine? I was formally introduced to Dr. Jennifer Amengual, my oncologist who specialized in lymphoma and is on the cutting edge of research into this area.

THE MIRACLE OF RELIEF
THE THIRD MIRACLE

Aesthetically all was beautiful in my purple room with a view, but my insides were being swallowed up by wild and fast-growing ugly cancer cells.

My oncology doctor stood before me to discuss my initial treatment plan.

I'm not sure how much I took in after she said the word chemotherapy, because at that point my head went right to my fear. "I'm a bit embarrassed and this may sound nutty to you but one of my biggest fears in going through chemo is throwing up," I said. "I'm terrified of going through nausea and vomiting throughout." To which Dr. Jen answered, "most people on this treatment cocktail don't have much of that, but you will have anti-nausea medication which I strongly advise you always take ahead of time. Don't wait until you feel that nausea come on; stay ahead of it and you'll be fine."

I, like Jerry Seinfeld states in one of his episodes, hadn't vomited in many years. I did not want chemo to ruin my record! Although he recalls the exact date on the show, I can remember the situation but not the year. I was out with hubby and another couple at a hotel club with dancing; the kind where you get on the small dance floor and move freely to some good old oldies. I started not feeling well and made it home on time to do the fearful deed which continued throughout the night – known by all as the 24 hour stomach virus.

The only activity this fear has curtailed is cruising. I had once been on a boat from Athens to the Greek islands in my late teenage years and was so nauseous the whole time that on the return trip I took extra Dramamine to knock me out so as not to feel anything. I still travel the world, just not on a boat. Although people tell me how much I'm missing out by not going on a cruise, I will not risk rocky waters to bring on such an awful feeling. I am perfectly happy with my travels sans cruising.

I felt a wee bit reassured by the doctor, but that picture of the sick cancer patient on the bathroom floor with her head in the toilet still loomed all too large in my mind. Too many movies floated that image across the forefront of my brain. Plus I've always had a fear of throwing up. Now it was taking on a life of its own.

Zofran, an anti-nausea medication, was to become my security blanket to which I held on tightly. And if I ever left home without a couple in a baggie, I'd almost become nauseous from anxiety over not having it with me. I would have loved to wear these small baby pills around my neck like those colorful candy necklaces, ready to swallow one if any hint of queasiness arose.

I listened to my doctor's advice and took one little guy every morning and one at bedtime.

As a non-medicine person, I'd have to feel really sick to take a Tylenol. And now here I was taking these pills prophylactically. But I was not about to risk the chance of my fear becoming a reality.

And so my record has continued on (maybe I should report that to Jerry!) and not only did I not throw up, I never got too nauseous. It is also quite amazing because as we know oftentimes we can worry ourselves into our fear where it becomes a reality.

This was truly a miracle! I let myself feel the wow of it at the end of my treatment. It warranted an unbelievable wow.

THE MIRACLE OF TOLERANCE
THE FOURTH MIRACLE

I have never been a medicine person. I have to be practically writhing in pain to take a Tylenol, and I start with the lowest amount to see if that does the trick, which it usually does. Except of course for antibiotics which have to be taken as directed. When I attempted a gummy (marijuana) for pain during my treatment, I cut it into a smaller piece to test my reaction. My head spun even with a quarter of that little guy. (And as far as those joyful-enhancing edibles, smokes, or drinks, I can become super silly without any help from those 'friends.')

Medicine has always been a last resort. I'm not sure how or why this came about. Say I have a high tolerance for discomfort and pain, I'm an au naturale person, I'm afraid of side-effects – both immediate and possible unknown long-term ones — I prefer putting less stuff into my body.

I've been able to deal more naturally with medical issues I've had throughout my life. My general doctors of first choice have been those with an integrative or functional approach.

My high cholesterol throughout my life was bestowed upon me by my thin father who was an avid and fast walker and didn't touch fried food until his 90s when he decided he would now eat his beloved french fries. He lived until 98 and only started taking pills at 92 when he had a stroke. I've dealt with mine as well with lifestyle measures, and it's basically remained the same with the good cholesterol number going up slightly. There is still more analysis into those numbers that should be done before automatically resorting to a pill.

I have osteoporosis which I've worked on naturally with more intake of green vegetables (no easy feat for me) and various forms of daily movement and targeted bone-strengthening exercises. Over the last few years my numbers have stayed the same. In this case maintaining is a positive. I've rejected taking life-long medicines or infusions for this.

When I had reflux and ulcers many years ago, after six weeks my integrative doctor took me off the routine medications for these conditions and put me on supplements and diet/life changes. Every morning hubby would end up on the lower part of the bed, having slowly slid down from the top incline under which cinder blocks had been placed to keep my head elevated; a helpful aid to reflux, along with a silly husband whose line was, "just put a rope around my neck and tie me to the top of the bed."

And when I had H-pylori, a gut bacteria that can cause a variety of stomach issues, knowing I could not tolerate a cocktail of about 10 antibiotics a day to knock it out, my integrative doctor put me on a regimen of supplements for a month, and lo and behold I tested negative when I was retested.

Of course there have been times when I had to take medicines. When I tested positive for TB after spending a year with my daughter Nava in two hospitals (when she had a life-threatening medical crisis), I had to take a specific antibiotic for many months, and I did well on it.

This was as opposed to the time I needed to take an antibiotic for a root canal, and I got C-diff from it. Then took another antibiotic to cure the C-diff only to end up in urgent care centers and an ER in Vancouver while on vacation. I could barely get dressed or shower as the joint pain was so debilitating, which made the hives and itchiness almost bearable. When I came home early from my trip and went to an allergist, I was given a note on his prescription pad which I still keep that says, 'serum sickness from clindamycin and vancomycin.' And although I was never tested as an adult, this has been added to my childhood allergic reaction of a rash and fever to penicillin.

And then there are those antibiotics that make me sick to my stomach which I can't manage.

So what's left in the antibiotic arsenal? I do fine with azithromycin, known as the Z pack, and with cipro.

Now when I need to take an antibiotic for my root canals and extractions of my lousy teeth, I am laughingly obliged with a Z pack, known to not be the drug-of-choice for teeth.

Thank G-d I have gotten through my life with no long-term medications. When I'd fill out medical forms in doctor's offices or anyplace else, I'd inevitably be asked, "Where are your medications?"

Oh, and I don't want to leave out the good reason for putting substances into me. (And no, it's not to get high.) I wasn't going to let malaria pills stop me from seeing my favorite animal up close and personal in its natural habitat – the beautiful and stately giraffe – on safari; and the wide-open land which belongs to all those beautiful creatures. Nor was a yellow fever shot going to stop me from going into the jungles of the Amazon and seeing the tribal ways of life. My college interest in cultural anthropology has permeated my life via leisure travel.

One of the reasons I was always afraid of getting sick was the idea of taking medicines and how I would be able to tolerate them.

Now comes cancer and here I am about to start having foreign and strong elements going into me, and a lot of pills to chug down each day. Three different antibiotics – antifungal, viral, and bacterial – were presented to me in a cup, along with a couple of other colorful pills. I laughed the first time a nurse brought them to me in the morning. What an assortment of pills and capsules, large and small, round and oblong/oval, that became my morning and nighttime routine. And even one of the antibiotics that I couldn't tolerate in the past, Dr. Jen had me take it every other day.

Usually I start one new pill at a time, waiting a couple of days to make sure I'm OK with it, before starting another new one, even with supplements. But now I was taking all of them together, not waiting to see if I had any negative side effects to any one.

I knew I couldn't play around with these, starting one at a time over a few days. There was no time. I was starting chemo and had to get these anti-everything pills into me. And so I started swallowing each one with trepidation hoping and praying they would sit well with me and do their job, protecting my body from any outside invaders that chemo might bring on. At least I was starting them before chemo so I could tease out, possibly, if I was having some negative reaction to a medication.

Perhaps the strong power of the mind over the body really worked here because....... lo and behold, I was fine with all of them! No stomach issues, no nothing.

Now that was truly miraculous for me!

THE MIRACLE OF ADAPTABILITY
THE FIFTH MIRACLE

Mmmmm, I can smell that coffee! The coffee that throughout my adult years I couldn't drink because it upset my all too easily-upsetting gut. It was a great churner in there until it sent me running to the bathroom. As a teen and young adult, Sanka and decaf cappuccinos were my coffee of choice. No pretty designs on the foam back then but thick yummy foam just the same of which I would eat some with a spoon and drink it while it formed a mustache around my lips.

Somewhere along the adult path of my life, I became unable to drink this strongly aromatic beverage that certainly captured my keen sense of smell. So I indulged my coffee flavor desire from other flavored things such as those hard candies known as Nips and coffee ice cream, the richest to me being Häagen-Dazs coffee chip. Perhaps it is no substitute for the real coffee deal, but it satisfied my coffee flavor love.

And so I became a tea drinker and a hot chocolate drinker. Wrapping my hands around a large funky mug of one of these two hot drinks totally satisfied me, and was a soothing and relaxing balm as a snack in the middle of the day or in the evenings. I was OK with these. My line became, *Yes, I love coffee, but it doesn't love me.* And so we parted ways for many years.

Until.....my cancer treatment. With each of my six rounds of chemotherapy, I had a lumbar puncture. Not a fun addition. It's basically a spinal tap where I got injected with Methotrexate as a preventive measure for cancer spread to the spine or brain. It was done as an outpatient procedure that took a few minutes. They find the right spot on the spine, wiggle that needle in and then put in the medicine. Each time I was taken into the procedure room the nurse would have to tell me to take deep breaths to slow down my anxiously fast breathing. I would always sit in the waiting area beforehand doing deep breathing. But getting into the room on that table, lying on my left side, would inevitably quicken my breath to numbers that brought the nurse's hand gently into mine. She would then instruct me to try to draw in slower breaths through my nose and out.

The aftercare was lying flat on my back for one hour, which was timed, in order to prevent headaches.

The first time I got this as an inpatient, since my whole first round of treatment was done over the course of five days in the hospital, I developed a scathing headache. I'm not someone who suffers with the usual migraine so I can't say I know what those headaches feel like, but this one was the worst I had ever felt. I couldn't talk, and I laid there with my eyes closed waiting for some medicine to kick in. I was given caffeine pills and told that every time I had this procedure I had to make sure I was drinking coffee. That seemed to be the thing to ward off those headaches. When I said I wasn't a coffee drinker, I was told to either become one or take the caffeine pills ahead of time.

With the encouragement of my coffee-drinking hubby, he started bringing a thermos of coffee with us on my days in the hospital for this lumbar puncture to begin my coffee experiment. I decided I would slowly try to see if I could tolerate some, starting with a few sips. Who knows, maybe after years my gut might've grown into some coffee tolerance. And sure enough…..

Each sip was fine. No cramping to send me into the bathroom. I was able to lay on the table having had about a quarter of a cup of coffee without much gut distress. A bubble here, a bubble there, but nothing to stop that delicious taste of coffee going down. And miracle of miracles….. no headaches for the next five rounds of lumbar puncture. My gut did its job of allowing the coffee to do its job.

So perhaps there are two miracles here: not even a hint of a headache after that first one, and becoming a coffee drinker.

I might add that this new tolerance of being able to drink coffee is a silver lining of this cancer treatment. Some good taste came out of this frequently distasteful experience.

I now enjoy my once-a-day morning coffee with my whipped-up coconut milk and cinnamon on top. I bought my own frother and excitedly look forward to this each morning. The foamier the better. But I haven't learned to make pretty curlicues on top, well not yet at least.

THE MIRACLE OF DEPENDABILITY
THE SIXTH MIRACLE

M y EPOCH treatment protocol was fixed at six rounds of 5-day infusions every 3 weeks — one week on, two weeks off — along with a lumbar puncture with an injection of chemo into my spine each cycle as a prophylactic measure.

After the first five-day round done in-hospital, the doctor suggested that I could continue my other rounds at home. I'd be hooked up to a small backpack that I'd carry around with me 24/7. I'd go to the hospital on Monday morning and get the bag of urine-like color chemo inserted into the pack. It was done in such a way that I'd be able to get my clothes, specifically my shirt, on and off with the bag intact, through my picc line on my left arm. This first bag lasted 48 hours. I'd go back on Wednesday to get a second bag to last another 48 hours and finish off the week on Friday when I'd return to get unhooked.

I felt a bit uneasy about all this. At least in the hospital I'm there if any problems arise with the actual infusions or with me. Dr. Jen calmly and comfortingly said she felt I was a good candidate for at-home treatment as I was basically in good, strong shape. Why be in a hospital room if I could be in the comfort of my home? Of course, she said the decision was mine. She continued to say I could try one round at home and if I don't like it or it doesn't go well, then I continue the next ones in-hospital. I wasn't signing my life away here with this decision. And if a problem arose with the apparatus, there was a number to call on the bag to trouble-shoot.

And so I decided I had nothing to lose to give it a shot. I went with her encouragement to do my second round at home, which then became my third, fourth, fifth and sixth. Yes, it went that well.

It was a bit inconvenient to say the least, like when going to the bathroom and making sure nothing got disconnected or entangled by accident. I was on a string and I had to stay within the confines of its length.

I learned to sleep flat on my back looking up at the ceiling, for fear of rolling onto my side. This was no easy feat for a cozy side-sleeper (as most of us are). I had to be very mindful of my sleeping position, which affected my sleep throughout the night. I didn't want to turn or mistakenly roll onto my left side where the hook-up was connected to my picc line on my left arm, and I didn't want to end up on my right side where the pull could be too taut and far. I was afraid of causing an inter-ruption in the flow or having it disconnect which immediately set off a beeping alarm. I climbed into bed gently and placed the bag close to me in bed like I was tucking in a dollie for a child, straightening out the tubes and patting it nice and neatly all around.

Beeping meant there was a stop in the flow usually signifying there was a tangle and I had to straighten or smooth out the tube. That didn't happen too often and when it did, it was a quick fix.

I walked around carrying this thing like you'd carry an egg in a box, making sure it didn't crack. Years ago, a high school project in health-ed was just this: carrying around an egg in a box for a week representing a baby and its fragility. This was not an easy task for a fast-moving person. I also had to be very intentional about this contraption, always making sure I didn't get too far from it. My fear of disconnecting was a looming presence, doing its best to keep me on a short leash.

The worst part was not being able to take a shower on Tuesday, Wednesday, Thursday and Friday. I'm a morning shower person and can't get dressed without first jumping into the shower. That early Monday morning shower had to last me the rest of the week, hopefully not a stinky one.

Getting unhooked on Friday early evening was a huge relief of freedom, and maybe even more than that, was knowing that a shower of the greatest appreciation was coming. That first shower of disconnection was delicious, as I stood there breathing in the heat and relaxation as the water poured down my back.

Fortunately, the only time something went truly amiss with the bag of chemo was shortly after leaving the hospital with my treatment in tow during the fifth cycle. It started beeping and wouldn't stop no matter what I did. We were still close to the hospital, and hadn't yet gotten onto the highway, so we turned around and went back to get it fixed. Phew — close call there.

And so my buddy bag and I worked well together at home for five rounds. I carried this appendage around with basically no interruptions. A great miracle it was.

THE MIRACLE OF FAITH AND TIMING
THE SEVENTH MIRACLE

As a Jew, I observe the Sabbath. It begins on Friday evening at sundown and ends on Saturday night when you can see three stars. It's basically a 24-hour day of rest and relaxation. Technically, it's the day God rested after His six days of creation. There is no work or travel, no technology, only the freedom of limits. Exactly because there are rules and limits to what can and can't be done, there is a freedom from the external, from the daily stresses and stressors of life. There's no load of laundry being thrown in, no phone calls, no computer or technology to be attached to, no errands to run. No piggy-backing appointments, no busyness, no hecticness.

This seventh day of rest is welcomed in with the lighting of the Sabbath candles on Friday evening. The candle-lighting time changes with the time of year; so during the summertime since the days are longer and it gets dark later, the candles are lit later.

Oftentimes I'm rushing to finish my Sabbath preparations, but once I light the candles, there is that Ahhh feeling of lightness and I plop down on the couch knowing that for the 24 hours there is nothing I am pulled to do. It's a time to be with one another with no distractions. There is a great psychological benefit – getting a forced interlude from the doings of life. We go to synagogue (shul), pray, eat two lavish meals – Friday night dinner and Saturday lunch – get together with family and friends, relax, nap, play games, take walks, read, and study the Bible.

Fridays ended my treatment for each round. I would get my last hour of a different medicine into me and then get unhooked from my chemo bag. What a feeling of freedom that was. I could move around freely and shower. The ease of life again without that hook-up matched the ease of welcoming in the Sabbath. But wait — I had to get home first, in time to light my candles. And getting home on time was no simple matter on a Friday early evening driving to Long Island. Summertime traffic going out to the hot spot of the Hamptons, and just general New York highway traffic was no rooftop open, hair blowing in the wind, singing aloud our 70's songs blasting on Sirius radio event. The creep-along traffic is the usual and customary. I would work at talking myself down to quell my stress at possibly missing the time to light my Sabbath candles.

All the timing was set from the get-go on Mondays with the first hook-up to the bag. It had to run 48 hours. I wanted to be done by about 4 o'clock so when I came back on Wednesday to get the next bag, that hook-up would also be completed by about 4. That way by Friday I'd get my next hour-long medicine, get flushed out and be out of the hospital by around 6 to get home in time to light candles. This was a computation of time all around. Timing was of the essence to bring in the Sabbath in a punctual way.

Nothing happens if I get home past the time to light my candles. I just wouldn't light. Serious health issues overtake everything. One of the Sabbath prohibitions is making a fire. So once the time of lighting passes, one can no longer light the candles. I have a good track record here — whether in the Amazon jungle or up in the Swiss mountains, I've always brought in the light of Sabbath at the correct time. There is a sanctity to time which is precious, and which brings in the warmth of light to soothe a busy, sick or traumatized soul.

Even when my daughter Nava was hospitalized for a year, on a ventilator for four months due to near-death complications from ulcerative colitis, I lit the Sabbath candles by turning on the switch of the candelabra that the hospital provided.

Most rounds I was out of the hospital by around 7 PM. That is cutting it very close to the lighting time of 8ish. Without much traffic it takes about an hour to drive in from my house to Columbia Presbyterian Hospital, which is in upper Manhattan in the Washington Heights area. I live in West Hempstead which is fairly close to the city line, not far out at all on Long Island. However, all the highways we take from the city to get home are the same ones that continue on out East to the Hamptons. Now add the Friday weekend traffic out East and that could easily be a two hour or more drive. I would calm myself down by thinking, "OK, I just won't light." Some things you can't control as much as you try, as good intentions as you have. I tried my best. All the nurses knew about Sabbath. I couldn't get the last medicine or the fluids to flush out the line into me at any faster rate.

The first time we left at 7 and got home just in time to light by 8. The Sabbath table was always set in advance, with my purple candelabra in place with the candles ready to be lit. Wow, it only took an hour! Where is the traffic going out east? It took us longer to get into the city in the morning.

And then the next round, and all rounds thereafter, completed on a Friday evening, I was home in time to light my candles. Miracle of miracles, I never missed a Friday night to bring in the Sabbath. I lit the candles with gratitude that I was able to light them. That truly beats all the odds of driving home with summer traffic on a Friday evening. Who knows, maybe because we left at 7 and not earlier it went so fast. Maybe all the traffic had gone out to Long Island earlier. Either way, it worked out for me, for something that strongly mattered. Something beyond simply no traffic was moving things along to get me home in a timely way to do what was important to me: to bring in the light and peace of the Sabbath after a difficult week of treatment. So I was able to welcome in my Sabbath in the way I always do, and I was able to bring in the light each and every Friday that completed that round of treatment. A miracle of light! A miracle of time!

THE MIRACLE OF MAINTENANCE
THE EIGHTH MIRACLE

"I'm driving to my best friend" is a joke in my family. One of numerous best friends, it could be my oral surgeon, gum dentist, crown dentist, root canal guy, or just general dentist. If I go a few months with no tooth problems, that's a win. Yes, I have lousy teeth. Since I was a child my mouth has been a silver mine, filled with huge fillings on almost every tooth, until some started breaking down as an adult and had to be repaired with a root canal and crown. Every time a new tooth problem reared its ugly head I'd get aggravated and eventually get to the point of, "at least it's fixable, it's not a disease."

Until it became a disease, and my newest tooth problem could not be fixed during treatment. Somewhere around my fourth cycle, one of my lovely lousy teeth cracked, and a piece of the large filling fell off. A very strict rule of Dr. Jen, my oncologist, was no dental work done during treatment. The mouth is a breeding ground for infection that could travel throughout the body. As an immuno-compromised person, this was a big NO for any type of dental work. The tooth actually wasn't bothering me so I let it be.

Until it DID start bothering me. And I called my general dentist and he said, "You have to come in to get it fixed so it doesn't get worse." To which I replied, "But I can't do any dental work." And we went back and forth for a bit and I started getting very upset.

This set me off into a tailspin of catastrophizing, high anxiety and sheer terror. What will be? What will I do? There didn't seem like there was any way to handle this problem. My teeth were tied! How do I leave it untreated, and yet I can't treat it? Friday night I was having a total meltdown of panic and thoughts of, "So this is what's going to do me in, my always fixable teeth except for now?"

After a bunch of calls to my numerous best friends, my oral surgeon said he'd come in to see me in his friend's dental office near me (instead of schlepping to his office in Brooklyn) on Saturday night.

Without putting too many instruments into my mouth, he took an x-ray and reassured me it wasn't infected. He spoke to my oncologist and together they decided on giving me a Z-pack (one of the antibiotics I can tolerate) prophylactically to hopefully help keep the tooth quiet. It would need to be treated as soon as I got the go-ahead from my oncologist, which would be at least two months later when I would hopefully be finished with chemo. With Dr. Ike's calm and caring manner, his reassuring hands cradling my head, and the results that the tooth wasn't bad, my anxiety level took a huge dive. I relaxed into my self-talk of 'hang on tooth for a bit, you can do it.' I prayed a lot over this guy, to stay OK for the time being.

And miracle of miracles, this tooth calmed down for the duration of my treatments. My mantra became: my teeth took care of me, so I must now take the best care I can of my teeth, never missing a brushing/flossing at night no matter how late it is, how sick or tired I feel.

When I was finally able to go to the root canal dentist, I was the happiest and most grateful camper to be sitting in that chair. Now who can say that about going to a dentist?!

THE MIRACLE OF PRECISION
THE NINTH MIRACLE

When I first met my oncologist and she discussed my treatment, she said in the best case scenario it would take about 4 ½ months to complete the six rounds of chemo. Meaning going straight through, every 3 weeks a new round, with no interruptions or breaks.

As we know, stuff happens, like cancer, seemingly out of the blue. How much more so when your body is getting toxicity pummeled into it; good to wipe out those nasty cancer buggers but not too good for the rest of the body. Blood counts can drop where it's dangerously low and therefore chemo has to be put off until the numbers go up, even a little. Infections can set in, anywhere in the body, putting off a chemo treatment for some time until the infection is treated and over.

I met many people in the hospital infusion waiting area with stories of delayed and dragged out treatment due to complications or bad enough side effects to hold off on a round. We can't begin to think about all the unknowns that the body can react to when dining on such a cocktail of toxicity.

Before each treatment, I'd have blood work done, wait to have it read, and then hope for the green light to proceed with the round of chemo treatment.

After three or four rounds, I had lost so much weight — over 20 pounds — that my anxiety level was through the roof. I'm a small person, always looking to gain some weight (although throughout my life the joke was, "Don't say that to too many people since they have the opposite problem!") I was terrified my body would not be able to withstand anymore treatment. It was being eaten away, along with the cancer cells, by what was being infused into it. It would break down and I would die or have to stop treatment altogether. How would my body stay strong enough to withstand this onslaught of toxicity? None of my 'tools' were working here to calm myself down and break the cycle of terror going on in my head. I went back and forth from catastrophizing over a possible terrible outcome to telling myself to stop thinking the worst. For the first time I asked to speak to a hospital therapist to see if they could help me get my head in a better place. I didn't get much from that discussion. My next call was to my {ex} sister-in-law Anny. She gave me the chizuk (strength) I needed to continue on in a bit of a better frame of mind. Her actual words are a blur now, but I got off the call feeling a bit more settled and on a less doom and gloom path. She had been a source of encouragement and strength to me during and after my divorce from her brother. And more recently she had cancer herself.

And so I stepped into the next round, surprised I was even allowed to continue, telling my body, 'you're more than half-way there, you can do this.'

Miracle of miracles, I completed my six rounds of treatment in the original time frame. No infections, no out-of-the-ordinary issues to necessitate a delay in treatment. My weight stayed steady at its low point. Although I needed a few blood transfusions by then, I was fine enough to continue treatment, eventually putting me into a 'no evidence of cancer' state.

THE MIRACLE OF IGNORANCE
THE TENTH MIRACLE

In the ER when I was told I had a large mass sitting on three organs I was also told I looked yellow; specifically my eyes were yellowish. I was jaundiced. "Had I not noticed?" the ER doctor asked me. "No, I didn't see that, nor did my husband." Apparently part of the large mass was sitting on my liver and was blocking and compressing my liver/bile ducts.

Just a couple of weeks prior, I had blood work done at a gastro visit because I wasn't feeling well and there was no indication with my liver numbers that anything was off. And now in the ER when they took blood, those numbers were off the chart.

After being admitted to the hospital that night, the first procedure I had - a sphincterotomy - two days later by an interventional gastroenterologist, entailed inserting two stents to open up the bile ducts, helping the bile to flow properly again.

They were to stay in for the duration of my treatment. They were a non-entity to me as I felt nothing. And they were never discussed again by my oncologist.

At my interim PET scan, at round four, they needed to see if the treatment was working. Those two stents were captured in the scan and partially blocked the scan pictures of that area. But my oncologist pretty much knew it was the stents and that the PET scan was good. The chemo was doing its job.

When treatment was completed and it was time for my post-treatment PET scan, it was discussed whether to have the stents removed before the scan. In the end, I'm not sure why, I had the scan first, noting the binary stents, and all was clear of lymphoma.

The following week I had my appointment with the doctor to remove the stents. Now here's the remarkable part.........

He said those stents are only in for 6-8 weeks due to higher risk of infection. If they must stay in longer, they're usually replaced. Ignorance is bliss. I knew nothing of this going into it.

I know now that they were left in because my oncologist didn't want any invasive procedures done during my treatment to avoid possible infection. This was like with my teeth where I had to wait until the chemo was done to have a root canal.

And so the miracle here is that my stents were in for six months – from before my chemo treatment started until after it all was completed — and there was no problem, no infection, no nothing. Had I known ahead of time about this usual shorter time frame, I would've been a nervous nelly, worrying about the what ifs each day that went by that they were still in me. Clearly everything is risk-assessed and prioritized when working to save a life.

In the darkness of the diagnosis and treatment, I am grateful that everything in my treatment worked out the best possible way according to plan. Taking note of these things working out well were my miracles and lit the way forward.

May you see the miracles in your everyday life and may they shine the light on your path.

PART TWO

PROFESSIONAL PROSPECTIVE AND COPING TOOLS

"Everything can be taken from a man but one thing: the last of the human freedoms—to choose one's attitude in any given set of circumstances, to choose one's own way."
~ *Viktor Frankl*

Existentialism and Logotherapy

Existentialism and specifically logotherapy is a large focus of my work, and life. These study the human condition from a more spiritual perspective, looking at meaning, purpose, value among other broader thoughts. As a near philosophy major in college, I am drawn to these areas of life study and enhancement. Dr. Viktor Frankl who survived numerous concentration camps during the Holocaust of WWII wrote his life-changing book, Man's Search For Meaning, soon after his miraculous freedom. In it he brings forth his concept of what he called logotherapy - the study of meaning and purpose. After reading this book back in my college years, and numerous times thereafter continuing to this day, always gleaning new bits of life-enhancing wisdom, the idea that we have a choice in how we handle and respond to our challenges has been profound for me. Whereas thinking, as many do, that it's our circumstances that determine the quality of our lives, it became a life-altering idea to me that our response to what happens to us is what shapes our lives. This has been my guiding light throughout my life. We may be a victim of circumstance but we can be empowered when we realize and buy into the idea that it is up to us in what we do with what befalls us, thereby not succumbing to a victim-like mentality. We have a choice in our response; and that can make all the difference in the world.

One of Dr. Frankl's patients famously said, "I broke my neck but it didn't break me." He went on to become a psychologist despite being paralyzed from the neck down. So similar to Christopher Reeve who went on to become even more impactful and influential after his tragedy of becoming paralyzed than in his role as superman. As he said, "A hero is an ordinary individual who finds the strength to persevere and endure in spite of overwhelming obstacles." It's what we do and how we respond to our greatest difficulties that shape our lives.

Personal Challenges: Cancer and Beyond

Cancer has been my biggest challenge yet; well, perhaps my second biggest, the first being finding out my second daughter, Nava, would have life-long disabilities. When I first heard the word cancer and for a few weeks thereafter I was numb. It wasn't until my lifelong close friend Eve said to me, "start using with yourself the tools you teach and use with your clients," that these core principles came alive in me. How was I going to handle and cope with my new adverse circumstance, with this awful and terrifying diagnosis and treatment? It was up to me; this part was in my purview of control. And Viktor Frankl's lifeline hit me right where it needed to, to get me out of my reverie of numbness and practical denial which itself is a {short term} coping strategy. I needed to take {some} control so I could cope with my new reality head-on.

I had a sense that I wanted some kind of therapy to support me along this journey, but not the typical kind of supportive counseling where you talk things out, emote and have a good listener on the other end. I had some good friends whom I could call on for that. I also instinctively knew, against the suggestions of many well-meaning people, that I did not want to attend a support group for people going through cancer. The last thing I wanted was to hear other people's horror cancer stories. I was frightened enough and thought that would just add to my fears and anxieties. I myself am a group facilitator and have led many various groups (not specifically cancer though) and right now did not at all aspire to the idea of misery loves company or that kind of support. And so as luck would have it, I found my therapist on a popular blog site that I frequent, Tiny Buddha. Elizabeth wrote a guest blog post on mindfulness, creativity and nature – all three things that resonate with me. Something bubbled up in me and felt so right that I reached out to her. Here was something different, something new and yes, creative that could help guide me on my path of treatment, supporting me in a more unique way. Although I'm only a stick-figure drawer and never thought of myself as artistic, maybe other forms of creativity could be awakened and kindled here. Something new, a unique distraction and maybe some new tools and insights along the way. And boy did my instinct serve me well. This turned out to be one of the best therapies I'd ever engaged in; and I've had my share of therapists over the years, for all different types of situations. I had a sense and an inner image that I had a lot of cobwebs in my chest/abdomen area (where the lymphoma was) that needed cleaning out; translated here as inner healing. With Elizabeth's training in Jungian theory and her artistry, it was a perfect combination of mandala-making together with insight and bringing forth some of the deep underlying webs of hurt and pain to work through.

The Creation of Coping Cards

I thought to create cards with pictures and quotes or wording to support me and give me strength as I was to begin my treatment. I love pictures - taking them and blowing up the beauties from my travels. I have a wall in my eclectic and fun den filled with these most memorable life-experiences. I also love quotes and sayings which I collect and have hung and pasted throughout my house. I combined both and it soon morphed into what I began calling my coping cards. Hubby would go to the local UPS center and get them laminated, and so my collection began.

My very first card was my mountain of strength which I took with me to the hospital and held in my hand during my first lumbar puncture. I focused on the mountain and visualized the strength of it coming into me. One of the medical people asked me about it to which I answered, "it's my visualization card." (before I thought of them as coping cards)

I did many more of them with Elizabeth where we wrote down intentions with each card - intentions of future outcomes, hopefulness, coping concepts. I continued making these cards even beyond my treatment, and into some of my emotional healing work around past issues of entanglement and pain.

Positive Psychology as a Framework

Another foundational part of my work, and personal life, is that of positive psychology. I did a certificate program with a master teacher, Tal Ben-Shahar, who taught one of the largest courses in Harvard on this subject. This too was life-changing. It helped enhance the quality of my life as a person and as a mental health professional. Positive psychology is the study of well being and human flourishing. Rather than only looking to alleviate pain and suffering, it looks to highlight and elevate human strengths and positive emotions towards life enhancement.

Tal Ben-Shahar states, "Things do not necessarily happen for the best, but I can choose to make the best of things that happen." This ties in with the concept of choosing our response to our circumstances. In fact a lot of basic tenets in positive psychology come from Viktor Frankl's logotherapy.

And so this whole framework of choice, of our responses to our difficulties, is a key part of who I've become. As my cancer started sinking in with the beginnings of treatment, my box of Dr. Frankl's concepts and those of positive psychology, became one that I opened frequently and started incorporating into my daily life. They were my coping tools and I became very intentional about using them.

Staying Present Amid Challenges

I knew I needed to keep calm and carry on. I wanted to stay present with each round of chemo and not spiral into anxiety about the upcoming ones and how I'd manage. As we know anxiety is fear and worry of the future. So staying present, which of course is a challenge in and of itself, was key. "I'm just dealing with round one now," I told myself. I would put up a mental STOP sign in my mind to try and prevent myself from ruminating and fretting about the next and the next rounds, and all the what if's. I visualized the big red sign with the bold letters and focused on the idea that "I'm focused on only this round now; let's do the best I can here and now and get through it."

Staying present was also greatly worked on with the help of my wonderful friend and meditation teacher, Eitan. He guided me over the phone through lots of beautiful healing visualizations. He had me close the light, sit up tall and begin to picture white/lavender/light pink light entering my body through the top of my head. Like a flashlight of light pastel colors, I envisioned it shining its light throughout my upper body, softening and healing the lymphoma, and keeping me in the here and now in a calming manner.

Finding Joy in Small Moments

They say it's the little things that make a difference. How true that is. Why wait for that once-in- a-blue-moon vacation or time to take that class or anything big that we so often put off for the 'right' time. We want to amplify our day-to-day life. Incorporating small bits of joy and pleasure into our week or even day can yield big results. From busy mommies who can't always be pouring from an empty cup, to stressed out and burned-out professionals who have no time for anything else, to caregivers who are juggling life on all ends, those small micro moments of enjoyment and reprieve can be replenishing and rejuvenating.

For me during my treatment, I intentionally sought out things/doings that made me feel good. So when my body wasn't pulling me down to sleep on the couch during the day or recline in my chair to take a nap by my sun-filled den doors, I watered my many plants, sat by my small and soothing waterfall in my backyard, and went around my garden cutting off the deadheads. And when I felt more energized, hubby and I went out to beautiful nature areas, walking a little and then sitting amidst the pretty greenery, flowers, ocean, woods. During the summer of my treatment, we discovered and explored many wonderful places on Long Island, marveling how much beauty there was in our own surrounding areas that we had never seen after living here for over 35 years. As we now know through science, nature is beneficial for our mental and physical health. As an overall, It is very calming, soothing and nourishing. I know I always feel better after being outside for a while; and even more so when amidst beauty.

These little outings made my day and week. Getting outside of myself and my illness, feeling something larger than myself in the natural world of the expansive ocean, the tall trees, the beautiful horizon at sunset, was a reprieve from sickness. I could take in and appreciate a larger life. Sunrises and sunsets took on a whole new level of grandeur.

Intentionally bringing in {small} pleasures into our lives on a regular basis yields positive emotions as well such as joy, love, curiosity, awe, and gratitude, all proven to boost our wellbeing.

I'm frequently updating my 'happiness boosters' list, adding in any new things of enjoyment I've discovered to put into my day or week. You might make your own fun list.

The Role of Color

A most enjoyable and fun thing I incorporated into each day was colors. I've always been a purple person. And although purple is still my all-time favorite color, I love the greens, blues and oranges as well. I have always stayed away from reds and pinks as I never thought they went with my red-haired, freckle-faced coloring. I grew up with my mom's colors being what I consider the boring ones: browns, grays, navys, beiges, blacks. Only later in life did she begin to add more colors to her wardrobe. In fact the one dress of hers that still hangs in my closet, that I can't get rid of 9 years after her death, is a rainbow colored silk suit. The one bold and vibrant color in my childhood home was a plush red velvet couch in the living room. I loved that cushiony sink-into comfy couch. Only recently have I been experimenting with red and pink - a pink pants outfit, a red scarf. I recently leased a white car with a red interior and I'm loving it. I smile every time I get into my car. Bringing forth my childhood years later on in life??!!

I had made the decision that I was not going to wear a wig; I didn't feel that was me. I decided I would wear scarves, bold and colorful ones. And so my daughters bought me bright scarves, solid and patterned, that I matched to each daily outfit. During Covid I had watched many videos on make-up for older women. I even had a couple of zoom make-up consultations. Eyeshadows became my thing as I learned how to apply more than one color on my lid at a time. Buying various colorful palettes became almost addictive as I now have so many large and small palettes of rich colorful eyeshadows, colors that I match daily with my clothing. Now during my illness, together with my hanger of numerous lively scarves, and my eye-enhancing shadows, I put together almost every day a colorfully fun Harriet-designed outfit. It lifted my spirits and made me feel more vibrant and alive. Not to mention it was a boost getting compliments from the hospital staff, always wondering what colors I would be in next.

Hair and Identity

I had my hair cut in three stages ahead of time, before it started falling out. I did not want to be holding clumps of fallen-out hair in the shower. My hair has been a defining feature throughout my life, both the color and the curls. On the more negative side, I certainly did not like being teased and called, "carrot top" and "freckle face" as a kid; and I wished for brown hair like everyone else and wanted to bleach off my freckles. But as I grew into my teenage years, I began to embrace my hair and love its color (the red had become more auburn) and natural curls. Those wanting-to-fit-in years where straight hair was the style, had me putting my hair up wrapped around an orange juice can to get it straight for the morning when I would still iron and tug it straight. Fast forward... raising three children thankfully got rid of that job and I started to go au naturale with my curls.

Because my hair held a lot of significance, I thought my hair loss and complete baldness would be a big deal for me. To my surprise it wasn't. To me it was a temporary issue that would resolve itself with time after the completion of treatment; new growth to be excited about. In the scheme of my fears, this was small potatoes.

Embracing the Full Spectrum of Emotions

As a therapist, I am obviously 'into' feelings and helping my clients feel and express theirs. As the saying goes, "we can't heal what we don't feel.' Permission to feel, as my teacher Tal Ben-Shahar says, is crucial to our well being. We need to allow ourselves to feel all our feelings, not only the 'good' ones. As he says, our feelings run through one main pipeline; if we shut off from the painful ones, we shut off from the positive ones as well. We are given a complete palette of emotions and we paint with them all to garnish that full, vibrant and whole life.

The 13th century poet, Rumi, has a beautiful poem called The Guest House, acknowledging all our feelings.

> **This being human is a guest house,**
> **Every morning a new arrival.**
> **A joy, a depression, a meanness,**
> **some momentary awareness comes**
> **as an unexpected visitor.**
> **Welcome and entertain them all!**
> **Even if they are a crowd of sorrows,**
> **who violently sweep your house**
> **empty of its furniture,**
> **still, treat each guest honorably.**

> He may be clearing you out
> for some new delight.
> The dark thought, the shame, the malice,
> meet them at the door laughing
> and invite them in.
> Be grateful for whatever comes,
> because each has been sent
> as a guide from beyond.

We know our society does not 'do' the difficult feelings too well. We are great at the quick fixes known as drinking and pill-popping; anything to numb us from feeling too much and too deeply those difficult and painful emotions. As someone who works with people grieving the loss of a loved one, too many run to their doctor for a pill to ease the pain of grief. Grief is not a sickness or something to be taken away with a pill; it is to be felt and gone through. The way out is through. And so the normalization of grief is in the teaching and helping people feel their natural and 'normal' sadness and pain. It seems counterintuitive but it is the way to come through it. As Brene Brown states so beautifully and simplistically in her Wholehearted Parenting Manifesto, "Together we will cry and face fear and grief. I will want to take away your pain, but instead I will sit with you and teach you how to feel it."

And so here I am with this illness upon me and I am not doing much of the feeling. There is grief due to illness too. Immediately, what came to my mind was that I was not going to let myself go to the 'why me' that spiraled me down years ago when I found out my daughter, Nava, would have life-long disabilities. Given a cancer diagnosis at 67, I was trying to embrace the 'why not me' thinking. It did take some work when my mind went to the people who don't take care of themselves, don't exercise, eat crap, and here I am doing all the 'right' lifestyle things and I get this. I did not want to go into this space that would bring me down and resentful.

When I was initially given the very grim preliminary finding in the ER, stone-like numbness set in, while hubby's faucet was turned on high. I tasted a few salty tears when I was admitted and brought up to my dark room at night and I laid in bed thinking about my life and simply not wanting it to be over yet. Although I felt greedy for thinking it - that I want more life, when so many die young {er}- I love the richness of my life and wanted to be privy to live into its beauty and adventure, continue connecting deeply in my work, and creating more fun and meaningful memories with my grand-kiddies and all who matter to me.

Action Mode: Coping Through Focus

Once biopsies and procedures began and I was given the correct and 'better' diagnosis, feelings seemed to go aside and action mode set in. In fact, I realized, and this became my metaphor, I was like a horse with blinders, putting one foot in front of the other and not looking here nor there, no side-ways to distract me from my task at hand. I did what I had to do to get through each cycle. I worked hard at keeping my anxiety at bay, yes, that's a feeling, and focused on keeping as good an attitude as possible. I didn't 'do' much sadness. When I talked to my close friends with whom I could be vulnerable, I didn't talk feelings. A couple of them commented on this too. I was more in my head, focused on being intentional and present, and working at coping each day.

I was doing what I needed to do and what would serve me well.

You could say that part of my 'horse with blinders' deal was something very unusual for me: I did not look anything up on Dr. Google. Curiosity is a big part of me, along with love of learning. They are what's considered two of my signature strengths. But in this case, they went by the wayside. I was too focused on going into all this in as untainted and unbiased way as possible; or one could say, in a minimally knowledge-able way. Again, so unlike me. I normally leave no stone unturned in my quest for knowledge and answers especially in challenging and difficult situations. I'm an asker and seeker. But in my case here, ignorance for me was bliss. Just follow along and step into the program. I was blindsided into this illness; I'll continue along blindfolded so as not to fuel my anxiety and flames of terror. I walked into the fire, hot coals under my feet, hopping from one to the other until I got to the final exit out. I did not want to see statistics, or read about side effects of my chemo cocktail and medications. I did not want to learn about probabilities of my type of cancer. In looking back now, I realize this was all part of my coping, to a sense with some denial. I didn't want to know too much. I usually want to know every crumb of information because as we know, knowledge is power. I left it all to my doctor and followed along with full trust in Dr. Amengual. She had come highly recommended as a leading researcher in my kind of cancer. Had I been given options for treatment, I would've done my due research. I felt no need to seek out other opinions or options.

Finding Silver Linings

I was very much focused on silver linings or as I like to say, the 'at leasts.' "At least it's summertime and I can be outside on my deck and people can visit me there," "if the bag of chemo had to beep, at least it was when we were still close to the hospital so we could get right back in a couple of minutes," "at least I was a good candidate for doing the chemo treatment at home and didn't have to be hospitalized for 5 days every round." This type of thinking kept me going fairly well. I want to add though that when someone else offers us a silver lining to our lousy situation or platitudes that usually start with 'at least,' it is not comforting or supportive. It can feel diminishing. But for me to see certain specifics as a lining filtering through some light, it kept me afloat and focusing on what was working well.

The Power of Gratitude

Gratitude is a researched-based concept that is a huge ingredient to well being and well living. When we shift our focus to the colorful and enticing pieces of yumminess on the top of our donut instead of honing in on the hole of emptiness in the middle, we shape our minds to start to notice and appreciate the good stuff around us. As Tal Ben-Shahar says, "when we appreciate the good, the good appreciates." When we come to a rosebush and we steer away from it because we are afraid of getting pricked by the thorns, we miss out on the beauty of the roses and their soft pedals. As opposed to stepping in with care in mind so we can get up close and take in their beauty . We then have not only enriched ourselves with their splendor but we are more attuned to other beauties around us. We start to see more of what we focus on.

There are some wonderful gratitude exercises that guide us towards seeing and appreciating the good and what we have in our lives even and especially through the difficult times. Even the pessimist can bump up his level by the smallest notch which makes a difference.

The 3 Blessings exercise is simply that: writing down three things we're thankful for. When done before bedtime, it helps shift our thinking away from the day's stresses and aggravations and hone in on even the smallest of goodness.

The WWW is another way of phrasing it, and no it's not a website: What Went Well or What's Working Well. Even in the throes of darkness and pain, to look for even the smallest things that are working well can be a great mindshifter. Documenting and focusing on these forms of gratitude help us cope as they are anchors to hold onto so that we don't drown in the depths of the dark waters. These are flickers of light dancing atop of the blackness.

And they don't have to be big. We don't have to wait for the good test result to feel thankful.

They can be the smallest seemingly inconsequential things: the ten minutes we got to just sit with a mug of hot chocolate with whipped cream on top and relax into the deliciousness of it; the great conversation we had with our friend; giving away a bag of clothing and hoping it adorns others well. Small daily things keep us on the path of more positive emotion. When things are going well, feeling gratitude for the ordinary keeps us from taking things for granted. We need the daily focus of the habitual as well, that brings us a sense of security and predictability, where we can breathe into that ah feeling of the 'working well' now.

MY COPING CARDS

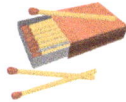

These cards, as I came to call them - my coping cards - focused me on going through and getting through my cancer journey. It became a creative and soothing way of capturing and visualizing, through pictures and words of intention, my hopes and process of coping through this time of difficulty. Creating them was therapeutic and calming, and provided me with glimmers of beauty and inspiration. Each card got laminated so they'd stay safe from spills and tears. I would take one, as I felt the need or mood, to the hospital; but mostly I used them at home, reading over and taking in the Intentions and enjoying the photos. And even more so, making them was the best and most beneficial part.

Creating something that resonates with you can be a powerful tool to help guide you through a challenging time and situation. For some it can be journaling, painting or coloring, or any form of personal expression. It serves as an outlet for hard and painful feelings, and as a representation of hope and intentions for the future, something to strive for.

THE CARD OF STRENGTH
CARD ONE

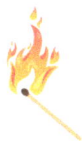

A visual of strength, the creation of this gave me a sense of empowerment over my situation. "I can handle this," although I was stepping into a scary new world of unknowns. Whether I was looking at it while waiting for my lumbar punctures or simply glancing at it at home by my bed, I was reminded of the harshness of nature's elements at times - thunder, lightning, and storms of all kinds - and that the mountainous terrain stays solid and strong. This was to be my symbol of stamina to hold onto. Against the backdrop of this mightiness, I was small but would be carried through by this everlasting creation of this strong force of nature.

Embracing Strength

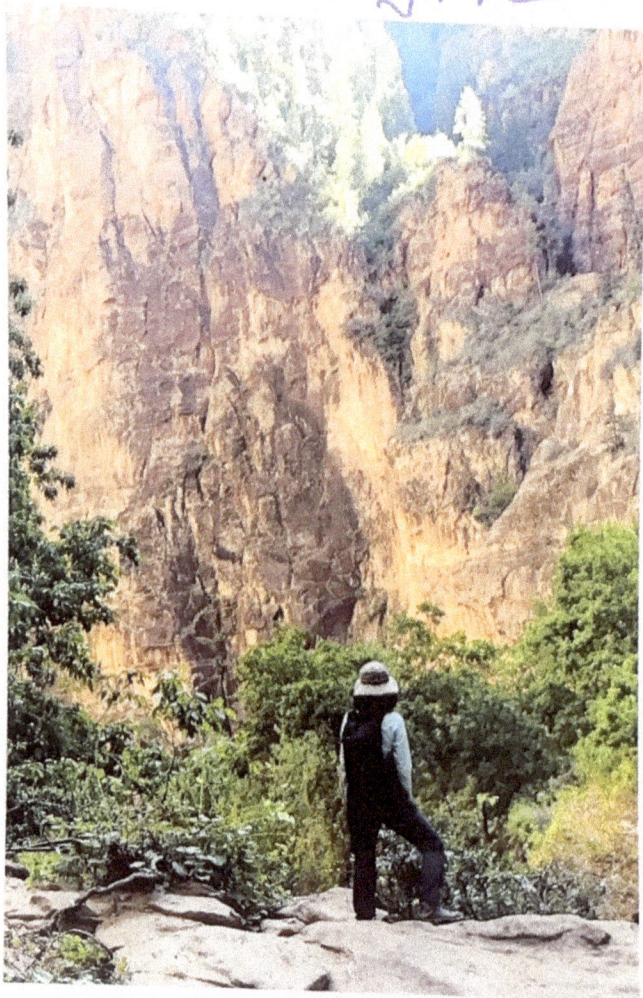

My intention is to
allow the strength
of the mountains to
support and
embrace me in
coping with this
process.

THE CARD OF HOPE
CARD TWO

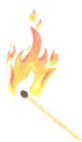

As a nature lover in all its beauty, I'm a gawker of sunsets. You might say I chase them. Wherever I am in my travels, I ask where to find the best sunset spot. Just ask my grandkids, always telling them to "come quick, look at this sky!" And in the car, "quick, turn around, look at the sunset behind you!" Perhaps when I'm gone, they will connect with me through these grandeurs of expansive color and keep Savta (grandma in Hebrew) close.

And of course sunrises awaken us to another day of life. I don't wake up often early enough to actually see the splashes of oranges slowly painting themselves across the expansive horizon, or the hints of color amidst the morning clouds, as the new day announces itself, but looking at this card by my bedside upon awakening, is a source of uplift as I step into a new day.

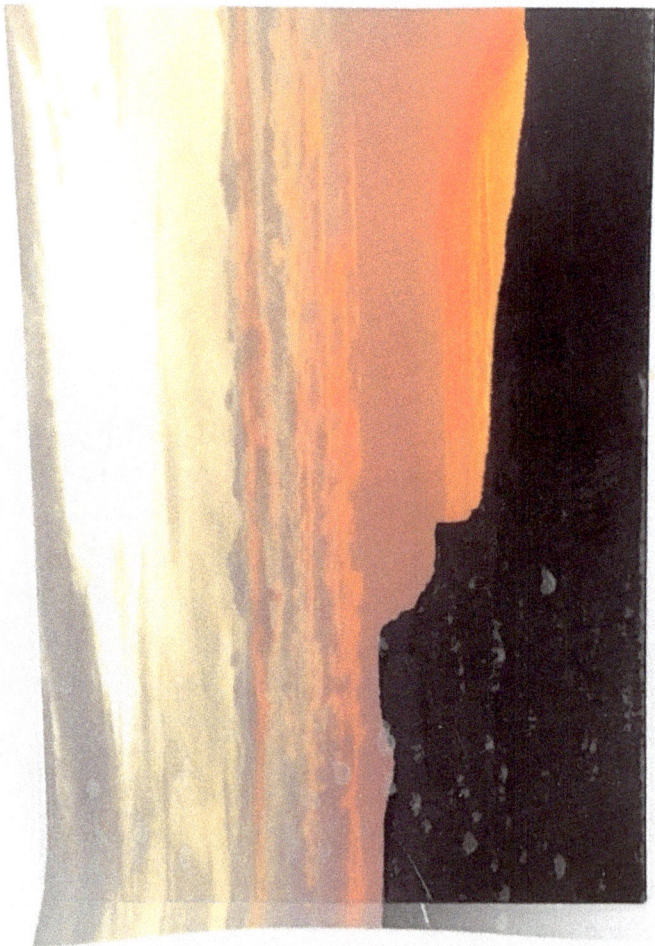

My intention is for the sunrise to support me in hope and optimism to meet the new day.

THE CARD OF FOCUS
CARD THREE

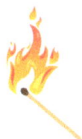

I realized I was going through my treatment putting one foot in front of the other, forging forward with each round of chemo. At some point the image of a horse with blinders came to me. There was no peripheral vision here: I was only looking and focused straight ahead. Just doing and following directives with what I had to do to get through the ordeal. Keeping on this linear path, heading straight for the finish line, was how I coped. A bit unusual for my normal coping style, but on this new terrain came this new way that even surprised me.

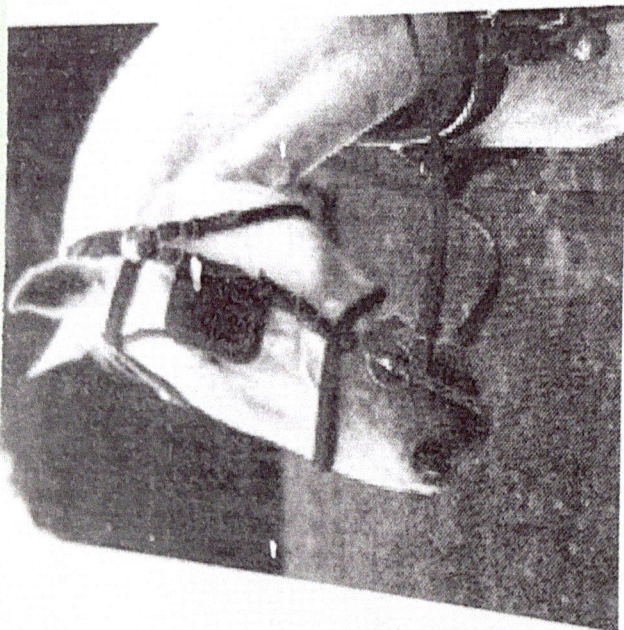

Putting one foot in front of the other

Like a horse with blinders

Keeping on the straight path

My intention is to be grateful for this aspect of myself that has served me well.

THE CARD OF PERSEVERANCE
CARD FOUR

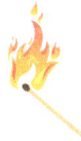

Through rough and steep terrain, I climb. I feel a sense of pride that I'm doing it; that I'm actually getting through each cycle of toxicity - killing off the bad guys and hopefully not doing too much damage to the good guys in there. I'm stepping through the possible poisonous snakes hiding underneath the rocks, looking down with each step for as good a solid footing as feasible, stopping periodically to look back and see how far I've come and what I've gotten through. Taking deep breaths along the way and moving on, not daring to look much to the sides, to those steep drops. For that opens up vistas of scary possibilities and just as the horse with blinders, I don't let myself go there.

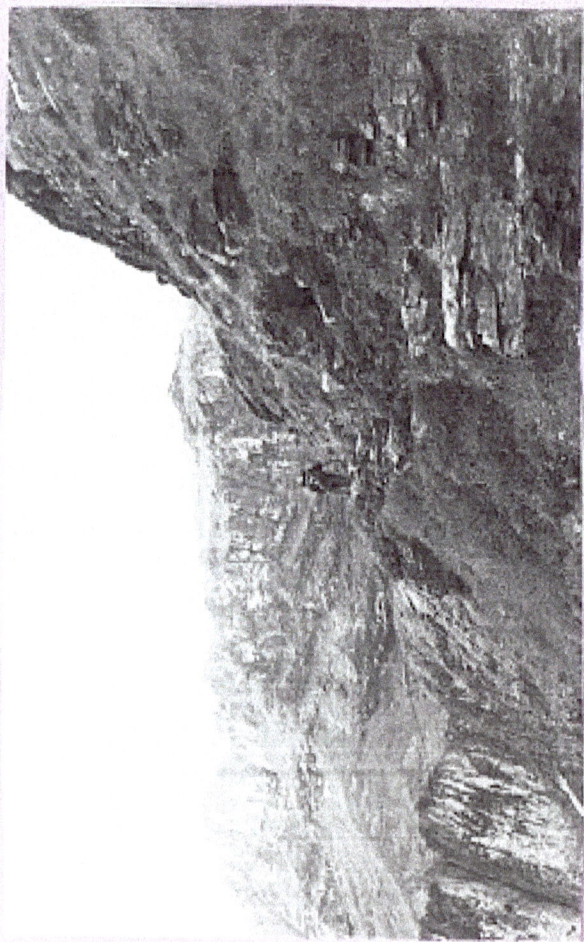

"I can't believe what I'm managing to Get Through

by Frank Bruni (The Beauty of Dusk)

My intention is to keep on climbing to the finish.

THE CARD OF FAITH
CARD FIVE

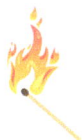

E very Friday evening at sundown I lit my Sabbath candles, miraculously on time each week, welcoming in the Sabbath, and more specifically at this time, appreciating the light after a challenging week. I was partnering to bring the light into me for a hopeful path forward. I lit my flames of gratitude for all that went well the past week, and for the strength to deal with it all in the best way possible. I hoped and prayed that they would cast their glow on my treatment journey for greater ease.

Sabbath candles
bringing in

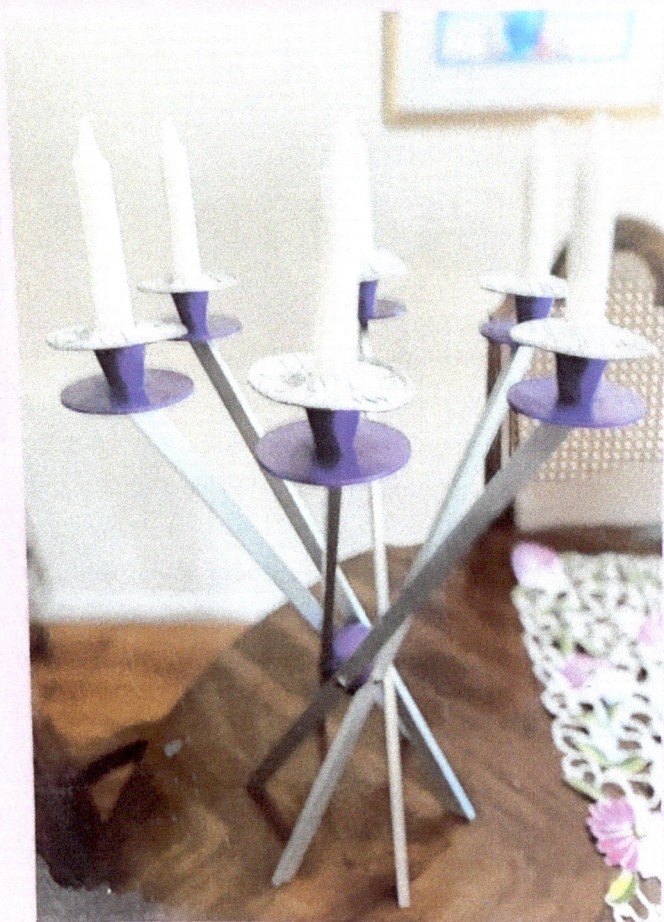

Gratitude for the
many miracles.

My intention is that the light of the weekly Sabbath candles be a perpetual reminder of the many miracles, large and small, during my treatment journey.

THE CARD OF SHRINKING
CARD SIX

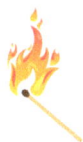

Meditating on my cancer shrinking became a clear and vivid visualization for me. To the point where I looked up (yes, utilizing Mr. Google's images, as opposed to my own photos), pictures of cancer cells getting smaller, and created a card for it. (And it was even purple!) We know there's a strong connection between the mind and body, not that thinking it makes it go away; but we also know there is power together with hope in visualizing a good outcome. Just think of the concept of the law of attraction. Some of it can seem hokey, but there is energy in what we put out there and how it effects us. What we focus on can either bring us down or lift us. That becomes a choice for us and can affect our coping.

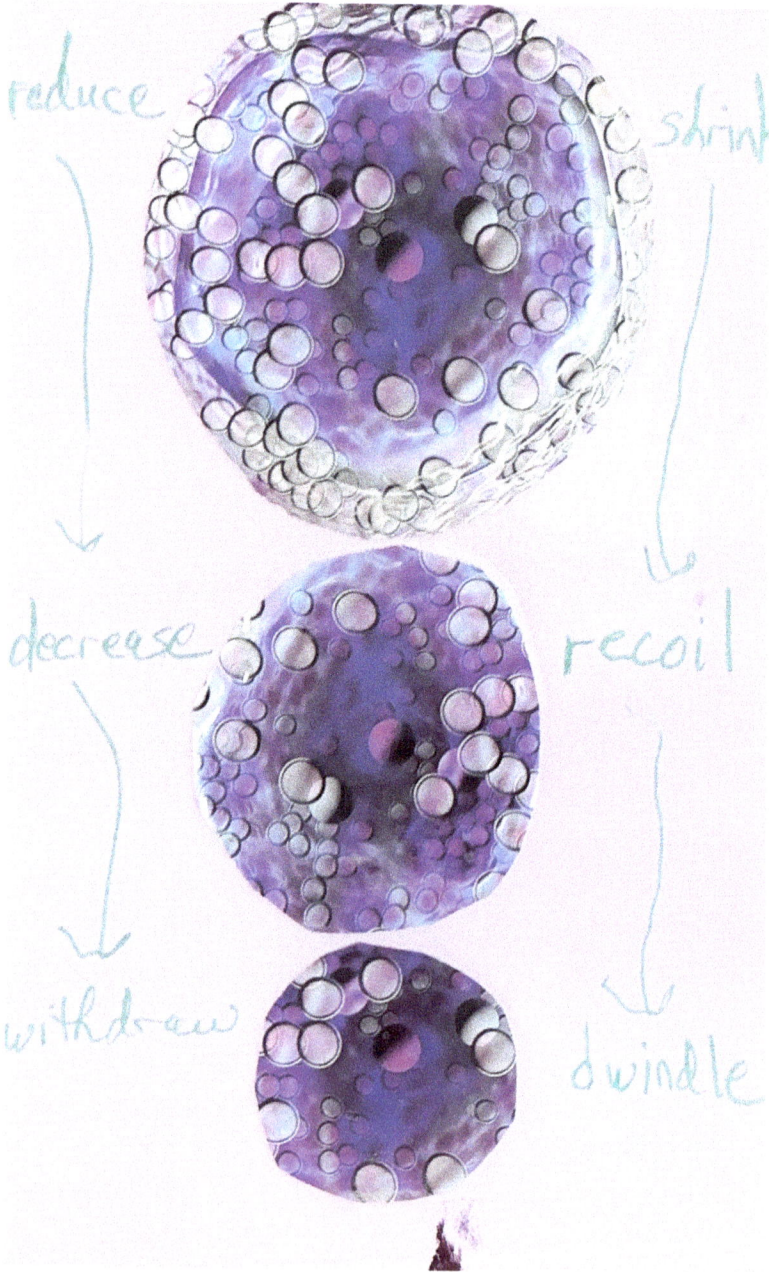

reduce

shrink

decrease

recoil

withdraw

dwindle

My intention is for
the cancer to be
shrinking

THE CARD OF GROWTH
CARD SEVEN

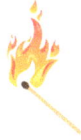

I knew when the hard knocks came to my door, I didn't want to just go through it (which is hard enough to get through), I wanted to grow through it. Of course coping was first and foremost, but keeping the growth factor in mind gave me something more to hold onto. That larger perspective helped keep me looking out and upward. There is something beyond the acuteness of my situation. A larger purpose.... Trying hard to maintain a strong base, while hoping to stretch higher.

Growth

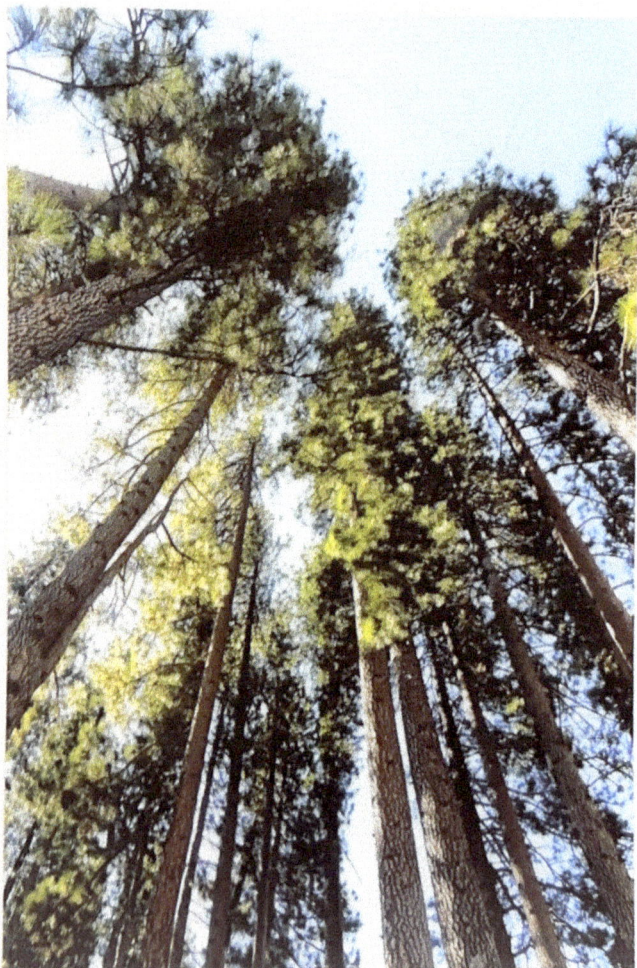

My intention is for these trees to support me in my ability to grow through this major challenge.

THE CARD OF EMERGENCE
CARD EIGHT

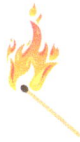

F ocusing on what was going well within the hardship of the treatment kept me somewhat in the line of light rays seeping through, with the goal being to come through the darkness into a bright and open clearing of sunlight. I held on to this image to keep me going. As much as I stayed very present to quell my anxiety, trying not to focus on the future, after round four I began to let myself envision actually coming through this. I visualized walking on a smooth path with the sunlight beaming down on me letting me know, 'You're back into the full beauty of life again; you've come through it well.'

From
Darkness

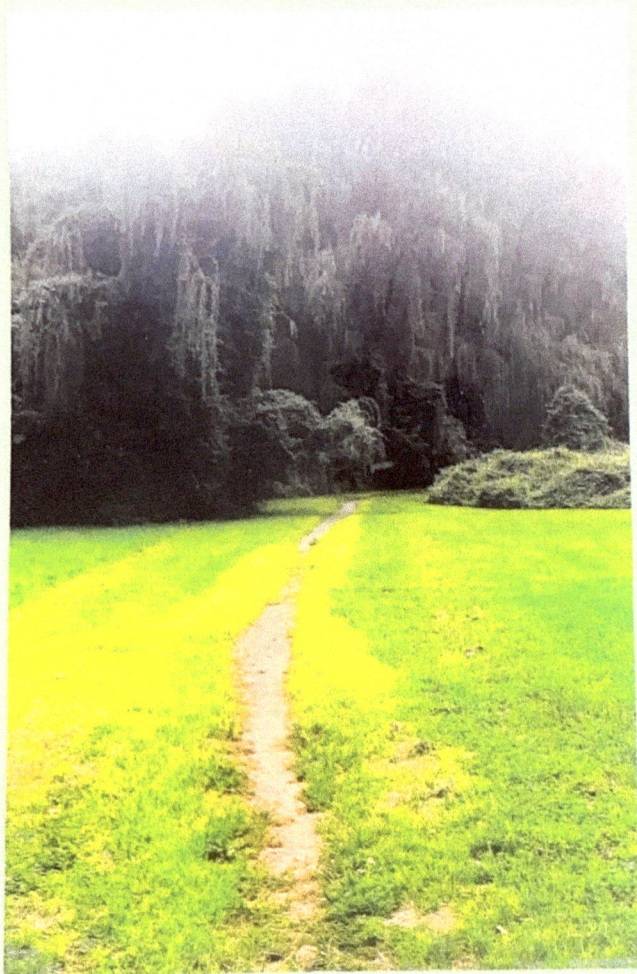

To
Light

My intention is to
restore my path
into the healing
light.

.

THE CARD OF HONOR
CARD NINE

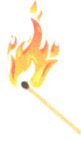

I n appreciation and awe of my body withstanding the onslaught of intense and shocking toxins to kill off the aggressively growing cancer, I am greatly motivated to work at giving back to it all the good stuff that it needs to repair itself and heal. I pledge to take care of it in my best way possible, nourishing and replenishing it with healthy choices. I feel indebted to my body for all the miracles it gave me and I want to reciprocate by inputting what it needs to continue healing.

Honoring your body

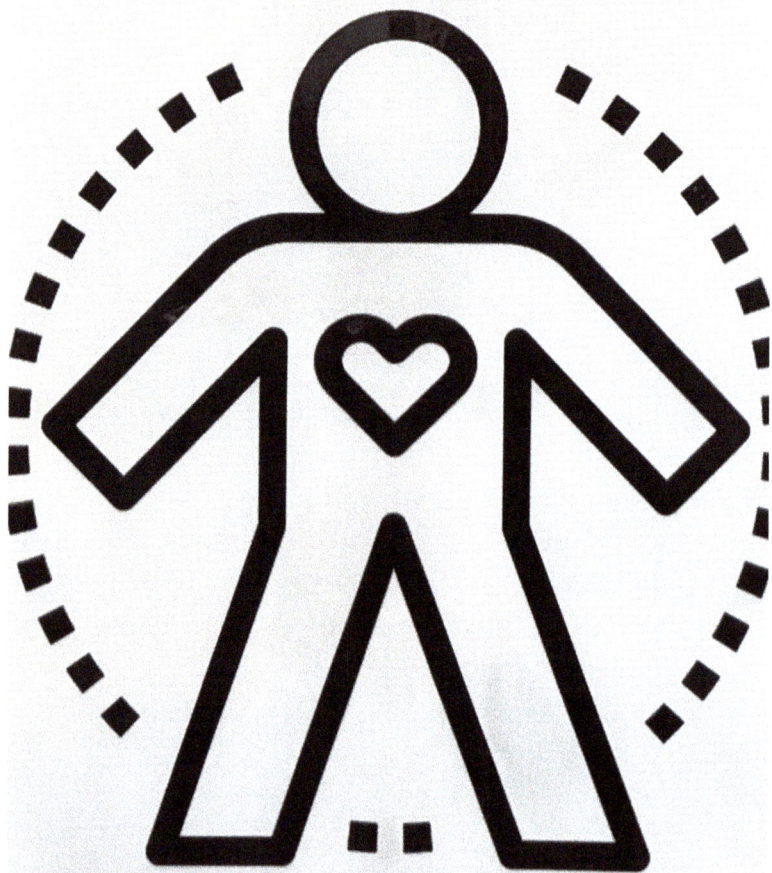

It took care of you;
now you take care of it.

My intention is to honor my body by giving it what it needs in the same way it has given me what I need to heal.

THE CARD OF GRATITUDE
CARD TEN

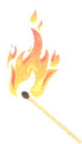

As I move beyond treatment, I am grateful to be looking at my path forward. My appreciation of the renewal of my life, the gift of my life, propels me to be open to paying it forward with more goodness and opportunities of service. "It's not what we expect from life, but rather what life expects from us." (Viktor Frankl) I feel that I owe life my best and welcome new chances to give back. When we are grateful for the good in our lives, we end up noticing more of it and we get more of it. It becomes an upward spiral. What we focus on becomes more of our reality.

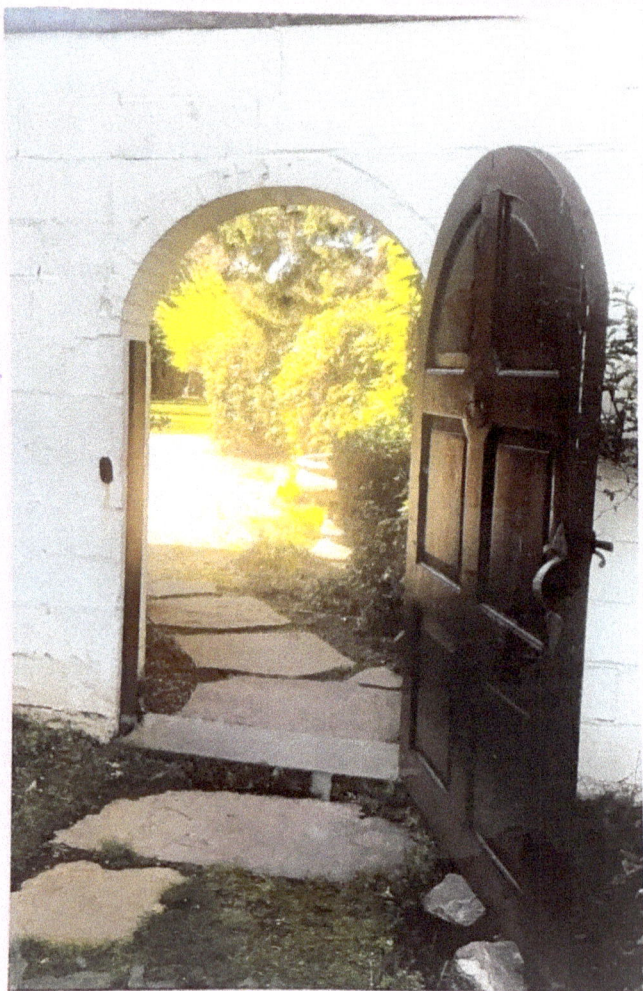

Gratitude

as I

begin my

path forward

My intention is to be grateful for and honor my journey/path forward as I remain open to the goodness and opportunities that reveal themselves.

GOING FORWARD

"If you have to go through hell, don't come out empty handed."
~ Rabbi Steve Leder

I truly believe that once we go through something difficult, that challenges our ability to get through, there is no going back to resuming our lives as before. We don't just pick up the pieces and continue. There is a whole new canvas of our lives that will by necessity evolve. We open ourselves up to it and work with a new reality. We may even crack open and do a deep spiral down but slowly we put ourselves back together, albeit in a new form. We can seek to use it as a springboard for our personal growth.

We are changed even if we don't yet recognize it in ourselves. We've utilized strengths we may never have known we had. We showed up in ways that may have surprised us, we carried on and wondered how we did it. Strengths lie dormant until called upon to come out.

When I was told I would have to learn to suction my daughter's trach, I said 'no way.' I had to walk out of the room when the nurses would do it for fear of my own gagging at the sound of the gurgles down in her throat. And yet when the time came for her home visits from the rehab hospital, I had to learn to do it. And so I did. I have carried that with me into the times since when I've said 'no way, I can't do that.' We take our struggles and alchemize them into new growth that adds a new layer of richness. They become new fibers of strength within us.

There is a beautiful art form known as kintsugi which has extended into a life philosophy. It is a Japanese form of art where a broken piece of pottery is glued back together with gold lacquer, making it look beautiful once again. Its fragility shows itself in the original crack, to which enhanced beauty is bestowed upon it with the new 'fixing' material.

Breaking down gives us the opportunity for repair, for major touch-ups. And we can grow back together in a newly worked-on version of ourselves. We can strut around with our beautified blemishes, marks and covered-over cracks with more pride, strength, wisdom and confidence. Nava wears her trach indentation in her throat as her badge of courage for all she endured and miraculously came through.

A beautiful quote from Hemingway: "The world breaks everyone and afterward many are strong at the broken places."

We as humans don't get fixed but we do heal. That is where the growth is – in how we come through and grow through our challenges and painful circumstances. This is our work: to use our struggles and pain in a positive way; otherwise what a waste of a 'good' adversity. We look to grow, heal and enhance our lives from it. Of course we never ask for hardships for self-transformation, but once they come in assaulting our lives, we can work to make something good from it, adding new meaning and purpose to our lives. Leonard Cohen has a beautiful line in his song, Anthem, "There is a crack, a crack in everything. That's how the light gets in."

There is a concept on the flip side of the coin of post-traumatic stress, known as post traumatic growth (PTG). It's the idea that one can experience positive change or growth after a struggle or adversity. This goes beyond resilience which is the ability to cope and adapt to difficulties and be able to bounce back from them. Some ways that post traumatic growth can be seen is through a greater appreciation of life, spiritual or religious change, assigning new meaning and purpose and enhanced relationships, and perhaps an overall different quality or essence to one's life. Knowing this idea, that we are not doomed to victimhood when coming out of a hard and lousy situation, that we can make some good out of bad, then we can lean into the idea that we can choose our way forward and create new quality to our lives. A well -lived life isn't one devoid of pain and adversity; it's one where we've weathered our struggles and weaved them into a new section of our life's tapestry; perhaps adding in more bold colors than before or blending more of the colors knowing that we can connect our pain and joy together.

When we know our values and what matters to us, we live more fully engaged as we lean into and prioritize what's important to us. We are more intentional about our choices and we realize we can choose to choose. We don't have to remain creatures of habit in everything we do.

I always remember when I suggested to a client upon her walking into my office that she sit in a different spot from her regular sink-in leather couch facing the desk. She resisted at first but upon a bit more prodding that this was actually a part of the therapy, she acquiesced and sat on a chair (not as comfy) giving her a different vantage point of the room. She noticed things she hadn't seen before: a picture of a gorgeous shade of turquoise ocean water, a plant dangling its long leaves over the bookcase, a door that opened into a bathroom. Voila – something new opened up here. The following week, to my surprise and amusement, she brought in a small pillow so she could sit on the chair more comfortably, for the time being in this new spot in the room. She thought it was so interesting that she saw things she hadn't noticed before. Stepping out of our habitual ways, changing things up, adds a quality of newness to our lives, which gets us more engaged, curious and interested.

Going forward in my post cancer life, means looking to pay forward the gift of my life. This incorporates tremendous gratitude and great appreciation for the renewal of my life, and always looking for ways to utilize my cancer in a positive way; adding value to the world around me. It's also living to the utmost after having banged heads up against mortality. We all know we have an end point but nothing brings it home more than a medical crisis. Our face gets pressed up against that window of mortality. Will the sun not rise any longer for us? And so when we get another chance at life, at living, we get to decide how we want to use our time in a more conscious, intentional way. We become active partners in our dance of life.

It means taking on more healthy ways of living that are cancer -resistant based. I feel more in control of my life when I'm doing my optimum at lowering my chances of recurrence. Ultimately, I believe that it's up to G-d and our lives are in His hands. But I put in my best efforts, which includes constantly learning new ways, ideas and concepts in the cancer world.

Cancer becomes a new chapter in my book of life. It does not define me. It does add a new layer of depth and meaning, and new growth. We are all individuals with many different circumstances occurring throughout our lives. How we use them, what we do with them, where we place them in the quilt of our lives, is what defines us. I view the boxes, large and small, as the specific areas and content, with the threads weaving them together, outlining and highlighting themes of growth and change, and ways of living that are the enhancements and connectedness displaying the richness of it all.

My wish is that I pay it forward well and do good in the space I occupy. "It is not what we expect from life, but rather what life expects from us." Viktor Frankl

ACKNOWLEDGMENTS

As soon as I put the idea of this book out there, in casual conversation, to Adrian Miller, networker extraordinaire, among her other gifts in content writing and business promotion, she connected me with the most encouraging and upbeat publisher, Stephanie Larkin, head penguin of Red Penguin Books. It took one minute on a zoom call to intuitively feel I was in the right hands. She 'got' me and my book project immediately. Talk about putting it out there and getting an immediate connection back. Synchronicity at its best!

So thank you Adrian for connecting me with Stephanie. Thank you Stephanie for being such an easy and pleasurable person to work with. Your encouragement and motivation every step of the way meant the world to me.

Hubby Alan, a support every step of the way. Every question, every fact check, he went to his files to immediately look up medical records for accuracy and times, and hard-to-look-back on specific information.

I am indebted to Dr. Myron Goldberg who got me the best oncologist for my type of cancer, and got me into Columbia Presbyterian hospital not a day too soon. I felt good and comfortable in the care of Dr. Jennifer Amengual, and NP's Supriya and Masoon, all so upbeat, calming and caring. They had faith in me and encouraged me all the way to the finish line.

From the time I was going through my treatment, my oldest grandson, Moshe, now almost 23, told me I had to write a book on my cancer journey. He would say to me, "Savta, you help people through so many things, now you can help people going through cancer." He was my biggest encourager. On so many of our calls (in Israel) he asked, "so, have you started your book yet," to which I answered "no, it's just not in me." Until I finished the book, Little Earthquakes by Sarah Mandel, and something shifted in me and I felt moved and inspired to begin to write my story, from both a personal and professional perspective, as Sarah Mandel did. I felt I had something to share. I was so excited to have Moshe be the first person I called to say that yes, I was now going to write my book. Every conversation since always includes, "how's the book coming?"

I am always blown away by my granddaughter Rachel's words, both in her writing and her speaking. I have a collection of her beautifully worded emails to me when I was sick, that I pasted onto cards and laminated for keepsake. She was then 11 years old. "...Even though you are sick you are still living a positive life, show'in it and rocking it. I know you will make it through no matter what because you're always ready for whatever comes your way. There aren't words to describe how much I love you times a million...."

My wonderful daughters, Esti, Nava and Penina are my treasures in my life and have made mommyhood the most meaningful 'career' of my life. They know I'd rather be anywhere but the kitchen; yet both Esti and Penina are cooks and bakers par excellence. I single out Penina here in appreciation (Esti lives in Israel) for being my amazing cook during the months of my treatment. When I couldn't eat much of anything, I ate her deliciously soothing chicken soup, vegetable soup and potato kugel. To this day, two and a half years post treatment, she continues to make them for me, plus more, for Shabbat meals.

I am truly grateful to my wonderful friends who were a constant support. From deeply connecting phone conversations, when I was up to it, to weekly Shabbat outdoor visits, to uplifting text messages, quotes, and emojis, to purple cozy and cute gifts, I felt embraced by my close friendships.

Special mention goes to Judi for her beautiful and yummy weekly fresh fruit platters, always with personal notes attached within the purple wrappings. And to my friend and her husband Eitan, who helped calm my nervous system with phone sessions of guided meditations and healing visualization, some of which I continue to use today on my own.

And specific thanks goes to Miriam S. for having Nava at her home for the religious holidays of Passover and Shavuot when I couldn't do much of anything.

To my great team of people helping me heal post-cancer: Dr. Miriam Rahav, trained in the metabolic approach to cancer, among many other areas of medicine, is a most warm, brilliant and beautiful healer. Her emphasis on wellness and working from the inside out is exceptional, especially in today's world of medicine.

I have changed much of my already healthy eating with the expert guidance of oncology nutrition consultant, Jen Nolan of Remission Nutrition. Her positive and gentle manner has encouraged me to go into the place I'd rather not spend much time in, but health calls and I admit I am doing a little more food preparation and experimentation, in the kitchen.

My trainer, Mitch Stein, who loves to say he saved my life by insisting (on the phone) I go to the ER that Sunday I came home from the boardwalk and was so upset that I was too weak to walk it. Six months later I went back to training with him and began his slow and sensitive training to rebuild my muscles and strength.

I am forever grateful to Elizabeth Bryan-Jacobs, my therapist, who in her beautifully creative, artistic and Jung-informed way brought a whole new experience into my life at a point when I desperately needed something to keep me afloat. And when my treatment was over, we really dove into the inner guck and worked on clearing out some of those entangled webs of pain.

I am uplifted by the Fred Astaire dance studio in Garden City, specifically Bryan, Ani and Eugene who brought me back to the exhilaration of dance life again. I had started dance lessons shortly before getting sick. I couldn't wait to get back to it and continue my bucket-list dream of learning to dance. And even being a part of some competitions. (not yet ready for dancing with the stars!)

My lifelong childhood friend, Miriam R. was recently taken from this world by one wrong step off the curb. She knew me better than most and was my cheerleader in my pursuits. She gave me the most honest feedback on my writing and I was therefore looking forward to her critique of sections of the book as I wrote them. I wanted her to see this book make its entry into the world. It is not to be. A framed photo of us sits by my computer, taken at my birthday party six months ago, where at least she got to hear my publicly spoken words of the impact she and our friendship had on me, as opposed to my words of eulogy at her funeral. For that I am grateful.

Every day I thank G-d for my life, for deciding to give me more time here.

ABOUT THE AUTHOR

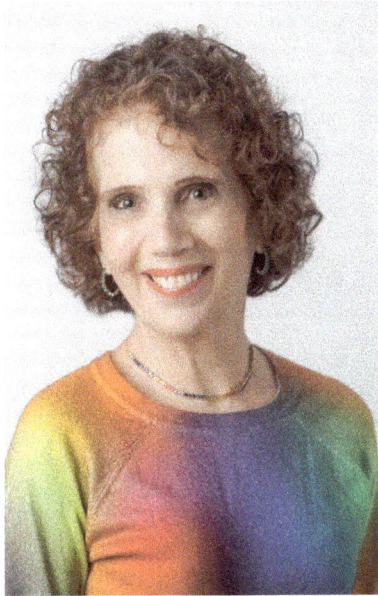

Harriet Cabelly is a seasoned grief counselor, therapist, speaker, and author dedicated to helping people navigate life's most challenging times. With decades of experience, Harriet has guided countless individuals through the complexities of grief, loss, and life transitions, providing support and tools to reclaim meaning and purpose.

A cancer survivor, Harriet brings both professional expertise and personal resilience to her work, offering a unique and compassionate perspective. As a mom and grandma, she understands the value of connection, love, and legacy, which shine through in her approach to helping others.

Harriet's passion lies in walking alongside those who feel overwhelmed by life's difficulties, empowering them to move forward with strength and hope. Her new book is a heartfelt guide for anyone seeking light in life's darkest moments, and is a testament to her belief that, even in pain, growth and healing are possible.

When she's not working with clients or speaking to audiences, Harriet cherishes time with her family, seeking out fun adventures, ballroom dancing, and traveling the world with her husband.

For more information, check out Harriet's website at rebuildlifenow.com and her previous book, *Living Well Despite Adversity*.